The ABZ of Vitamins And Minerals

Earl Mindell

Arlington Books
King Street, St. James's
London SW1

THE ABZ OF VITAMINS & MINERALS

First published 1988 by
Arlington Books (Publishers) Ltd
15–17 King Street, St James's
London SW1
Reprinted 1988
Reprinted 1990

Reproduced from The Vitamin Bible
by Earl Mindell, also published by
Arlington Books

Typeset by Wordbook Ltd, London
Printed in England by Clays Ltd, St Ives plc

British Library Cataloguing in Publication Data

Mindell, Earl
ABZ of vitamins & minerals.
1. Minerals in human nutrition   2. Vitamins
in human nutrition
I. Title
613.2′8   TX553.M55

ISBN 0-85140-724-4

Introducing Vitamins

What Vitamins Are

We must obtain vitamins from organic foods, or dietary supplements in order to sustain life. When I mention the word "vitamin", most people think "pill". Thinking "pill" brings to mind confusing images of medicine and drugs. Though vitamins can and certainly often do the work of both medicine and drugs, they are neither.

Quite simply, vitamins are organic substances necessary for life. Vitamins are essential to the normal functioning of our bodies and, save for a few exceptions, cannot be manufactured or synthesised by our bodies. They are necessary for our growth, vitality, and general well-being. In their natural state they are found in minute quantities in all organic food. We must obtain them from these foods or in dietary supplements.

Supplements, which usually come in pill form and around which so much controversy has arisen, are still just food substances, and, unless synthetic, are also derived from living plants and animals.

It is impossible to sustain life without all the essential vitamins.

Vitamins are neither pep pills nor substitutes for food. A lot of people think vitamins can replace food. They cannot. In fact, vitamins cannot be assimilated without ingesting food. There are a lot of erroneous beliefs about vitamins, and I hope this book can clear up most of them.

Vitamins are not pep pills and have no calorie or energy value of their own.

Vitamins are not substitutes for protein or for any other nutrients, such as minerals, fats, carbohydrates, water — or even for each other!

Vitamins themselves are not the components of our body structure.

You cannot take vitamins, stop eating, and expect to be healthy.

If you think of the body as a car's combustion engine and vitamins as spark plugs, you have a fairly good idea of how these amazing minute food substances work for us. Vitamins regulate our metabolism through enzyme systems. A single deficiency can endanger the whole body. Vitamins are components of our enzyme systems which, acting like spark plugs, energise and regulate our metabolism, keeping us tuned up and functioning at high performance.

Compared with our intake of other nutrients like proteins, fats, and carbohydrates, our vitamin intake [even on some megadose regimens] is minuscule. But a deficiency in even one vitamin can endanger the whole human body.

The A B Z of Vitamins

Vitamin A

Facts

Vitamin A is fat soluble. It requires fats as well as minerals to be properly absorbed by your digestive tract.

It can be stored in your body and need not be replenished every day.

It occurs in two forms — preformed vitamin A, called retinol [found only in foods of animal origin], and provitamin A, known as carotene [provided by foods of both plant and animal origin].

Vitamin A is measured in USP Units [United States Pharmacopoeia], IU [International Units], and RE [Retinol Equivalents].

7,500 IU daily is the maximum adult dosage.

What it can do for you

Counteract night blindness, weak eyesight, and aid in the treatment of many eye disorders. [It permits formation of visual purple in the eye].

Build resistance to respiratory infections.

Shorten the duration of diseases.

Keep the outer layers of your tissues and organs healthy.

Promote growth, strong bones, healthy skin, hair, teeth, and gums.

Help treat acne, impetigo, boils, carbuncles, and open ulcers when applied externally.

Aid in the treatment of emphysema and hyperthyroidism.

Deficiency disease

Xerophthalmia, night blindness.

Best natural sources

Fish liver oil, liver, carrots, green and yellow vegetables, eggs, milk and dairy products, margarine, and yellow fruits.

Supplements

Usually available in two forms, one derived from natural fish liver oil and the other water dispersible.

Water-dispersible supplements are either acetate or palmitate and recommended for anyone intolerant to oil, particularly acne sufferers.

Vitamin A acid [retin A] is sometimes prescribed for acne, but is available only by prescription. 10,000 to 25,000 IU are the most common daily doses.

Toxicity

More than 100,000 IU daily can produce toxic effects in adults, if taken for many months.

More than 18,500 IU daily can produce toxic effects in infants.

Toxicity symptoms include hair loss, nausea, vomiting, diarrhoea, scaly skin, blurred vision, rashes, bone pain, irregular menses, fatigue, headaches, and liver enlargement.

Enemies

Polyunsaturated fatty acids with carotene work against vitamin A unless there are antioxidants present.

Personal advice

You need at least 10,000 IU vitamin A if you take more than 400 IU vitamin E daily.

If you are on the pill, your need for A is *decreased*.

If your weekly diet includes ample amounts of liver, carrots, spinach, sweet potatoes, or cantaloupe, it's unlikely you need an A supplement.

Do not supplement your dog's or cat's diet with vitamin A unless a vet specifically advised it.

Vitamin B1 (Thiamine)

Facts

Water soluble. Like all the B-complex vitamins, any excess is excreted and not stored in the body. It must be replaced daily.

Measured in milligrams [mg.].

B vitamins are synergistic — they are more potent together than when used separately. B1, B2, and B6 should be equally balanced [i.e. 50 mg. of B1, 50 mg. of B2, and 50 mg. of B6] to work effectively.

The official RDA for adults is 1.2 to 1.4 mg. [During pregnancy and lactation 1.4 mg. is suggested.]

Need increases during illness, stress and surgery.

Known as the "morale vitamin" because of its beneficial effects on the nervous system and mental attitude.

Has a mild diuretic effect.

What it can do for you

Promote growth.
Aid digestion, especially of carbohydrates.

Improve your mental attitude.

Keep nervous system, muscles, and heart functioning normally.

Help fight air or seasickness.

Relieve dental post-operative pain.

Aid in treatment of herpes zoster.

Deficiency disease

Beriberi.

Best natural sources

Dried yeast, rice husks, whole wheat, oatmeal, peanuts, pork, most vegetables, bran, milk.

Supplements

Available in low-and high-potency dosages — usually 50 mg., 100 mg., and 500 mg. It is most effective in B-complex formulas, balanced with B2 and B6. It is even more effective when the formula contains antistress pantothenic acid, folic acid, and B12. 100 to 300 mg. are the most common daily doses.

Toxicity

No known toxicity for this water-soluble vitamin. Any excess is excreted in the urine and not stored to any degree in tissues or organs.

Rare excess symptoms include tremors, herpes, oedema, nervousness, rapid heartbeat, and allergies.

Enemies

Cooking heat easily destroys this B vitamin. Other enemies of B1 are caffeine, alcohol, food-processing methods, air, water, oestrogen, and sulpha drugs. [See page 92].

Personal advice

If you are a smoker, drinker, or heavy sugar consumer, you need more vitamin B1.

If you are pregnant, nursing, or on the pill you have a greater need for this vitamin.

As with all stress conditions — disease, anxiety, trauma, post-surgery — your B-complex intake, which includes thiamine, should be increased.

Vitamin B2 [Riboflavin]

Facts

Water soluble. Easily absorbed. The amount excreted depends on bodily needs and may be accompanied by protein loss. Like the other B vitamins it is not stored and must be replaced regularly through whole foods or supplements.

Also known as vitamin G.

Measured in milligrams [mg.]

Unlike thiamine, riboflavin is *not* destroyed by heat, oxidation, or acid.

For normal adults, 1.2 to 1.6 mg. is the RDA. Slightly higher amounts are suggested during pregnancy and lactation.

Increased need in stress situations.

America's most common vitamin deficiency is riboflavin.

What it can do for you

Aid in growth and reproduction.

Promote healthy skin, nails, hair.

Help eliminate sore mouth, lips, and tongue.

Benefit vision, alleviate eye fatigue.

Function with other substances to metabolise carbohydrates, fats, and proteins.

Deficiency disease

Ariboflavinosis — mouth, lips, skin, genitalia lesions.

Best natural sources

Milk, liver, kidney, yeast, cheese, leafy green vegetables, fish, eggs.

Supplements

Available in both low and high potencies – most commonly in 100 mg. doses. Like most of the B-complex vitamins, it is the most effective when in a well-balanced formula with the others. 100 to 300 mg. are the most common daily doses.

Toxicity

No known toxic effects.
Possible symptoms of minor excess include itching, numbness, sensations of burning or prickling.

Enemies

Light — especially ultraviolet light — and alkalis are destructive to riboflavin [Opaque milk cartons now protect riboflavin that used to be destroyed in clear glass milk bottles.] Other natural enemies are water [B2 dissolves in cooking liquids], sulpha drugs, oestrogen, alcohol. [See page 92.]

Personal advice

If you are taking the pill, pregnant, or lactating, you need more vitamin B2.
If you eat little red meat or dairy products you should increase your intake.

There is a strong likelihood of your being deficient in this vitamin if you are on a prolonged restricted diet for ulcers or diabetes. [In all cases where you are under medical treatment for a specific illness, check with your doctor before altering your present food regimen or embarking on a new one.]

All stress conditions require additional B complex.

Vitamin B6 [Pyridoxine]

Facts

Water soluble. Excreted within eight hours after ingestion and, like the other B vitamins, needs to be replaced by whole foods or supplements.

B6 is actually a group of substances — pyridoxine, pyridoxinal, and pyridoxamine — that are closely related and function together.

Measured in milligrams [mg.].

Requirement increased when high-protein diets are consumed.

Must be present for the production of antibodies and red blood cells.

There is some evidence of synthesis by intestinal bacteria, and that a vegetable diet supplemented with cellulose is responsible.

The recommended adult intake is 1.6 to 2.0 mg. daily, with higher doses suggested during pregnancy and lactation.

Required for the proper absorption of vitamin B12.

Necessary for the production of hydrochloric acid and magnesium.

What it can do for you

Properly assimilate protein and fat.

Aid in the conversion of tryptophan, an essential amino acid, to niacin.

Help prevent various nervous and skin disorders.

Alleviate nausea [many morning-sickness preparations that doctors prescribe include vitamin B6].

Promote proper synthesis of antiaging nucleic acids.

Reduce night muscle spasms, leg cramps, hand numbness, certain forms of neuritis in the extremities.

Work as a natural diuretic.

Deficiency disease

Anaemia, seborrhoeic dermatitis, glossitis.

Best natural sources

Brewer's yeast, wheat bran, wheat germ, liver, kidney, heart, cantaloupe, cabbage, blackstrap molasses, milk, eggs, beef.

Supplements

Readily available in a wide range of dosages — from 50 to 500 mg. — in individual supplements as well as in B-complex and multivitamin formulas.

To prevent deficiencies in other B vitamins, pyridoxine should be taken in equal amounts with B1 and B2.

Can be purchased in time-disintegrating formulas that provide for gradual release up to ten hours.

Toxicity

No known toxic effects.

Possible symptom of an oversupply of B6 is night restlessness and too vivid dream recall.

Enemies

Long storage, canning, roasting or stewing of meat, water, food-processing techniques, alcohol, oestrogen. [See page 92.]

Personal advice

If you are on the pill, you are more than likely to need increased amounts of B6.

Heavy protein consumers need extra amounts of this vitamin.

If you are taking a B complex, make sure there is enough B6 in the formula to be effective. B6 is expensive, and some vitamin formulas are short on it. If you can't remember your dreams, it might be that you need a separate pyridoxine tablet in addition to your multi-vitamin or B complex.

Vitamin B12 [Cobalamin, Cyanocobalamin]

Facts

Water soluble and effective in very small doses.

Commonly known as the "red vitamin", also cyanocobalamin.

Measured in micrograms [mcg.].

The only vitamin that contains essential mineral elements.

Not well assimilated through the stomach. Needs to be combined with calcium during absorption to benefit body properly.

Recommended adult dose is 3 mcg., with larger amounts suggested for pregnant and lactating women.

A diet low in B1 and high in folic acid [such as a vegetarian diet] often hides a vitamin-B12 deficiency.

A properly functioning thyroid gland helps B12 absorption. Symptoms of B12 deficiency may take more than five years to appear after body stores have been depleted.

What it can do for you

Form and regenerate red blood cells, thereby preventing anaemia.

Promote growth and increase appetite in children.
Increase energy.
Maintain a healthy nervous system.
Properly utilise fats, carbohydrates, and protein.
Relieve irritability.
Improve concentration, memory, and balance.

Deficiency disease

Pernicious anaemia, brain damage.

Best natural resources

Liver, beef, pork, eggs, milk, cheese, kidney.

Supplements

Because B12 is not absorbed well through the stomach, I recommend the time-release form of tablet so that it can be assimilated in the small intestine.

Supplements are available in a variety of strengths from 50 mcg. to 2,000 mcg.

Doctors routinely give vitamin-B12 injections. If there is a severe indication of deficiency or extreme fatigue, this method might be the supplementation that is called for.

Daily doses most often used are 5 to 10 mcg.

Toxicity

There have been no cases reported of vitamin-B12 toxicity, even on megadose regimens.

KITCHEN CUPBOARD REMEDIES

BOILS

A BREAD and milk poultice helps draw pus from a boil. Soak two slices of bread in milk, mash, and then wrap in gauze. Apply to the boil for half an hour.

EARACHE

OLIVE oil can loosen ear wax. Lie on your side and put a few drops in your ear, then sit up. Using garlic-infused oil (not actual pieces) may help prevent infection.

washed their hands.

The American-developed technology uses sensors in a bedside monitor to detect soap fumes.

If it picks up the smell on staff hands, it flashes green. But if does not, it vibrates and buzzes, reminding staff to wash their hands.

The monitor, called HyGreen, is designed to reduce the risk of infections spreading.

Hospital-acquired infections are estimated to kill at least 5,000 people a year in the UK.

As well as the monitor, medical staff can wear a badge that registers the exact time they squirt soap or gel from the wall-mounted dispenser.

This means hand-washing patterns can be downloaded on to a computer and analysed by infection control specialists.

---

ergic rhinitis.

of the vegetable is being given to
with the condition, which is
by inflammation of the nasal
(symptoms include a chronic
throat and blocked nose).
initis is both triggered and
ted by pollution.

rial, a small amount of fluid
g diesel exhaust particles will
d into the patients' noses.
nt is equivalent to the diesel
omeone living in a big city
le over the course of two
atients will then drink a cup of
tract to test its effect.
own to contain high levels
e, which enhances
tory enzymes,' say the
searchers.

Enemies

Acids and alkalis, water, sunlight, alcohol, oestrogen, sleeping pills. [See page 92.]

Personal advice

If you are a vegetarian and have excluded eggs and dairy products from your diet, then you need B12 supplementation.

Combined with folic acid, B12 can be a most effective revitaliser.

Surprisingly, heavy protein consumers may also need extra amounts of this vitamin, which works synergistically with almost all other B vitamins as well as vitamins A, E, and C.

Women may find B12 helpful — as part of a B complex — during and just prior to menstruation.

Vitamin B13 [Orotic Acid]

Facts

Unavailable in the United States, and not recognised as a vitamin in the United Kingdom.

Metabolises folic acid and vitamin B12.

No RDA has been established.

What it can do for you

Possibly prevent certain liver problems and premature ageing.

Aid in the treatment of multiple sclerosis.

Deficiency disease

Deficiency symptoms and diseases related to this vitamin are still uncertain.

Best natural sources

Root vegetables, whey, the liquid portion of soured or curdled milk.

Supplements

Available as calcium orotate in supplemental form.

Toxicity

Too little is known at this time to establish guidelines.

Enemies

Water and sunlight.

Personal advice

Not enough research has been done on this vitamin for recommendations to be made.

Vitamin B15 [Pangamic Acid]

Facts

Not recognised as a vitamin in the United Kingdom.

Water soluble.

Because its essential requirement for diet has not been proved, it is not a vitamin in the strict sense.

Measured in milligrams [mg.].

Works much like vitamin E in that it is an antioxidant.

Introduced by the Russians while the U.S. food and Drug Administration has doubts about it.

Action is often improved by being taken with vitamins A and E.

What it can do for you*

Extend cell life span.

Neutralise the craving for liquor.

Speed recovery from fatigue.

Lower blood cholesterol levels.

Protect against pollutants.

*U.S. research in the case of B15 has been limited. The list of benefits given here is based on my study of Soviet tests.

Aid in protein synthesis.
Relieve symptoms of angina and asthma.
Protect the liver against cirrhosis.
Ward off hangovers.
Stimulate immunity responses.

Deficiency disease

Again, research has been limited, but indication
point to glandular and nerve disorders, heart disease
and diminished oxygenation of living tissue.

Best natural sources

Brewer's yeast, whole brown rice, whole grains
pumpkin seeds, sesame seeds.

Supplements

Usually available in 50-mg. strengths.
Daily doses most often used are 50 to 150 mgs.

Toxicity

There have been no reported cases of toxicity
Some people say they have experienced nausea on
beginning a B15 regimen, but this usually disappear
after a few days and can be alleviated by taking the

B15 supplement after the day's largest meal.

Enemies

Water and sunlight.

Personal advice

Despite the controversy, I have found B15 effective and believe most diets would benefit from supplementation.

If you are an athlete or just want to feel like one, I suggest one 50-mg. tablet in the morning with breakfast and one in the evening with dinner.

An important supplement for residents of big cities and high-density pollution areas.

Vitamin B17 [Laetrile]

Facts

Not recognised as a vitamin in the United Kingdom.

One of the most controversial "vitamins" of the decade.

Chemically a compound of two sugar molecules [one benzaldehyde and one cyanide] called an amygdalin.

Known as nitrilosides when used in medical doses.

Obtained from apricot pits.

One B vitamin that is not present in brewer's yeast.

Touted as a cancer treatment in most of the United States at this date and legal in fifteen states but rejected by the Food and Drug Administration on the grounds that it might be poisonous due to its cyanide content.

What it can do for you

It is purported to have specific cancer-controlling and preventative properties.

Deficiency disease

May lead to diminshed resistance to cancer.

Best natural sources

A small amount of laetrile is found in the whole kernels of apricots, apples, cherries, peaches, plums, and nectarines.

Supplements

Daily doses most often used are .25 to 1.0 g.

Toxicity

Though no toxicity levels have been established yet, taking excessive amounts of laetrile could be dangerous. Cumulative amount of more than 3.0 g. can be ingested safely, but not more than 1.0 g. at any one time.

According to the Nutrition Almanac, five to thirty apricot kernels eaten through the day, but never all at the same time, can be a sufficient preventive amount.

Personal advice

There is now extensive literature available on laetrile. I strongly advise personal research and a consultation with a physician before embarking on any regimen involving B17.

Biotin [Coenzyme R or Vitamin H]

Facts

Water soluble, and another fairly recent member of the B-complex family.

Usually measured in micrograms [mcg.].

Synthesis of ascorbic acid requires biotin.

Essential for normal metabolism of fat and protein.

The RDA for adults is 150 to 300 mcg.

Can be synthesised by intestinal bacteria.

Raw eggs prevent absorption by the body.

Synergistic with B2, B6, niacin, A, and in maintaining healthy skin.

What it can do for you

Aid in keeping hair from turning grey.
Help in preventive treatment for baldness.
Ease muscle pains.
Alleviate eczema and dermatitis.

Deficiency disease

Eczema of face and body, extreme exhaustion, impairment of fat metabolism.

Best natural sources

Nuts, fruits, brewer's yeast, beef liver, egg yolk, milk, kidney, and unpolished rice.

Supplements

Biotin is usually in most B-complex supplements and multiple-vitamin tablets.
Daily doses most often used are 25 to 300 mcg.

Toxicity

There are no known cases of biotin toxicity.

Enemies

Raw egg white [which contains avidin, a protein that prevents biotin absorption], water, sulpha drugs, oestrogen, food-processing techniques, and alcohol. [See page 92.]

Personal advice

If you drink a lot of eggnogs made with raw eggs you probably need biotin supplementation.

Be sure you're getting at least 25 mcg. daily if you are on antibiotics or sulpha drugs.

Balding men might find that a biotin supplement may keep their hair there longer.

Vitamin C [Ascorbic Acid]

Facts

Water soluble.

Most animals synthesise their own vitamin C, but man, apes, and guinea pigs must rely upon dietary sources.

Plays a primary role in the formation of collagen, which is important for the growth and repair of body tissue cells, gums, blood vessels, bones, and teeth.

Helps in the body's absorption of iron.

Measured in milligrams [mg.].

Used up more rapidly under stress conditions.

The RDA for adults is 45 mg. [higher doses recommended during pregnancy and lactation].

Recommended as a preventive for crib death or sudden infant death syndrome [SIDS].

Smokers and older persons have a greater need for vitamin C. [Each cigarette destroys 25 mg.]

What it can do for you

Heal wounds, burns, and bleeding gums.

Accelerate healing after surgery.

Help in decreasing blood cholesterol.

Aid in preventing many types of viral and bacterial infections.

Act as a natural laxative.

Lower incidence of blood clots in veins.

Aid in treatment and prevention of the common cold.

Extend life by enabling protein cells to hold together.

Reduce effects of many allergy-producing substances.

Prevent scurvy.

Decrease infections by 25 percent and cancers by 75 percent if taken in 1,000-mg. to 10,000-mg. daily dosage, according to Dr. Linus Pauling.

Deficiency disease

Scurvy.

Best natural sources

Citrus fruits, berries, green and leafy vegetables, tomatoes, cauliflower, potatoes and sweet potatoes.

Supplements

Vitamin C is one of the most widely taken supplements. It is available in conventional pills and effervescent tablets, time-release tablets, syrups, powders and pastilles.

The form that is pure vitamin C is derived from corn dextrose [though no corn or dextrose remains.]

The difference between "natural" or "organic" vitamin C and ordinary ascorbic acid is primarily in the individual's ability to digest it.

The best vitamin-C supplement is one that contains the complete C complex of bioflavonoids, hesperidin, and rutin. [Sometimes these are labelled citrus salts.]

Tablets and capsules are usually supplied in strengths up to 1,000 mg. and in powder form sometimes 5,000 mg. per tsp.

Daily doses most often used are 500 mg. to 4 g.

Rose hips vitamin C contains bioflavonoids and other enzymes that help C assimilate. They are the richest natural source of vitamin C. [The C is actually manufactured under the bud of the rose — called a hip.]

Toxicity

No proven toxic effects, though excessive intake might cause unpleasant side effects in specific cases. Occasional diarrhoea, excess urination, kidney

stones, and skin rashes may develop on megadoses
Cut back dosage if any of these occur.

Enemies

Water, cooking, heat, light, oxygen, smoking
[See page 93.]

Personal advice

Because vitamin C is excreted in two to three
hours, depending on the quality of food in the
stomach, and it is important ot maintain a constant
high level of C in the bloodstream at all times
I recommend a time-release tablet for optimum
effectiveness.

If you're taking over 750 mg. daily, I suggest a
magnesium supplement. This is an effective deterrent against kidney stones.

Carbon monoxide destroys vitamin C, so city
dwellers should definitely up their intake.

You need extra C if you are on the pill.

I recommend increasing C doses if you take aspirin
or simply want your other vitamins to work better.

If you take ginseng, it's better to take it three
hours before or after taking vitamin C or foods high
in the vitamin.

Calcium Pantothenate [Pantothenic Acid, Panthenol, Vitamin B5]

Facts

Water soluble, another member of the B-complex
family.

Helps in cell building, maintaining normal growth, and development of the central nervous system.

Vital for the proper functioning of the adrenal glands.

Essential for conversion of fat and sugar to energy.

Necessary for synthesis of antibodies, for utilisation of PABA and choline.

The RDA [as set by the FDA] is 10 mg. for adults.

Can be synthesised in the body by intestinal bacteria.

What it can do for you

Aid in wound healing.

Fight infection by building antibodies.

Treat post-operative shock.

Prevent fatigue.

Reduce adverse and toxic effects of many antibodies.

Deficiency disease

Hypoglycaemia, duodenal ulcers, blood and skin disorders.

Best natural sources

Meat, whole grains, wheat germ, bran, kidney, liver, heart, green vegetables, brewer's yeast, nuts, chicken, crude molasses.

Supplements

Most commonly found in B-complex formulas in a variety of strengths from 10 to 100 mg.

10 to 300 mg. are the daily doses usually taken.

Toxicity

No known toxic effects.

Enemies

Heat, food-processing techniques, canning, caffeine, sulpha drugs, sleeping pills, oestrogen, alcohol. [See page 92.]

Personal advice

If you frequently have tingling hands and feet, you might try increasing your pantothenic acid intake — in combination with other B vitamins.

Pantothenic acid can help provide a defence against a stress situation that you forsee or in which your are involved.

1,000 mg. daily has been found effective in reducing the pain of arthritis, in some cases.

Choline

Facts

A member of the B-complex family and a lipotropic [Fat emulsifier].

Works with inositol [another B-complex member] to utilise fats and cholesterol.

One of the few substances able to penetrate the so-called blood-brain barrier, which ordinarily protects the brain against variations in the daily diet, and go directly into the brain cells to produce a chemical that aids memory.

The RDA has not yet been established, though it's estimated that the average adult diet contains between 500 and 900 mg. a day.

Seems to emulsify cholesterol so that it doesn't settle on artery walls or in the gallbladder.

What it can do for you

Help control cholesterol build up.

Aid in the sending of nerve impulses, specifically those in the brain used in the formation of memory.

Assist in conquering the problem of memory loss in later years.

Help eliminate poisons and drugs from your system by aiding the liver.

Produce a soothing effect.

Deficiency disease

May result in cirrhosis and fatty degeneration of liver, hardening of the arteries, and possibly Alzheimer's disease.

Best natural sources

Egg yolks, brain, heart, green leafy vegetables, yeast, liver, wheat germ, and, in small amounts, in lecithin.

Supplements

Six lecithin capsules, made from soya beans, contain 244 mg. each of inositol and choline.

The average B-complex supplement contains approximately 50 mg. of choline and inositol.

Daily doses most often used are 500 to 1,000 mg.

Toxicity

None known.

Enemies

Water, sulpha drugs, oestrogen, food-processing, and alcohol. [See page 92.]

Personal advice

Always take choline with your other B vitamins.

If you are often nervous or "twitchy" it might help to increase your choline.

If you are taking lecithin, you probably need a chelated calcium supplement to keep your phosphorus and calcium in balance, since choline seems to increase the body's phosphorus.

.Try getting more choline into your diet as a way to a better memory.

Vitamin D [Calciferol, Viosterol, Ergosterol, "Sunshine Vitamin"]

Facts

Fat soluble. Acquired through sunlight or diet. [Ultraviolet sunrays act on the oils of the skin to produce the vitamin, which is then absorbed into the body.]

When taken orally, vitamin D is absorbed with fats through the intestinal walls.

Measured in International Units [IU].

The RDA for adults is 400 IU.

Smog reduces the vitamin-D-producing sunshine rays.

After a suntan is established, vitamin-D production through the skin stops.

What it can do for you

Properly utilise calcium and phosphorus necessary for strong bones and teeth.

Taken with vitamins A and C it can aid preventing colds.

Help in treatment of conjunctivitis.

Aids in assimilating vitamin A.

Deficiency disease

Rickets, severe tooth decay, osteomalacia, senile osteoporosis.

Best natural sources

Fish liver oils, sardines, herring, salmon, tuna, milk and dairy products.

Supplements

The maximum permitted daily dose in the United Kingdom is 400 IU.

Usually supplied in 400 IU capsules, the vitamin itself is derived from fish liver oil.

Daily doses most often taken are 400 IU.

Toxicity

2,500 IU daily over an extended period of time can produce toxic effects in adults.

Dosages of over 5,000 IU daily might affect some individuals adversely.

Signs of toxicity are unusual thirst, sore eyes, itching skin, vomiting, diarrhoea, urinary urgency, abnormal calcium deposits in blood-vessel walls, liver, lungs, kidney and stomach.

Enemies

Mineral oil, smog. [See page 92.]

Personal advice

City dwellers, especially those in areas of high smog density, should increase their vitamin-D intake.

Night workers, nuns, and others whose clothing or life-style keeps them from sunlight should increase the D in their diet.

Children who don't drink D-fortified milk should increase their intake of D.

Dark-skinned people living in northern climates usually need an increase in vitamin D.

Do not supplement your dog's or cat's diet with vitamin D unless your vet specifically advises it.

Vitamin E [Tocopherol]

Facts

Fat soluble and stored in the liver, fatty tissues, heart, muscles, testes, uterus, blood, adrenal and pituitary glands.

Formerly measured by weight, but now generally designated according to its biological activity in International Units [IU].

Composed of compounds called tocopherols. One of the eight tocopherols — alpha, beta, gamma, delta, epsilon, zeta, eta, and theta — alphatocopherol is the most effective.

An active antioxidant, prevents oxidation of fat compounds as well as that of vitamin A, two sulphur amino acids, and some vitamin C.

Enhances activity of vitamin A.

The U.S. RDA for adults is 30 IU.

60 to 70 percent of daily doses are excreted in faeces. Unlike other fat-soluble vitamins, E is stored in the body for a relatively short time, much like B and C.

Important as a vasodilator and an anticoagulant.

Products with 25 mcg. of selenium for each 200 units of E increase E's potency.

What it can do for you

Keep you looking younger by retarding cellular ageing due to oxidation.

Supply oxygen to the body to give you more endurance.

Protect your lungs against air pollution by working with vitamin A.

Prevent and dissolve blood clots.

Alleviate fatigue.

Prevent thick scar formation externally [when applied topically — it can be absorbed through the skin] and internally.

Accelerate healing of burns.

Working as a diuretic, it can lower blood pressure.

Aid in prevention of miscarriages.

Deficiency disease

Destruction of red blood cells, muscle degeneration, some anaemias and reproductive disorders.

Best natural sources

Wheat germ, soya beans, vegetable oils, broccoli, Brussels sprouts, leafy greens, spinach, enriched flour, whole wheat, whole-grain cereals, and eggs.

Supplements

Available in oil-base capsules as well as water-soluble dry-base tablets.

Usually supplied in strengths from 100 to 1,000 IU. The dry form is recommended for anyone who cannot tolerate oil or whose skin condition is aggravated by oil.

Daily doses most often used are 200 to 2,000 IU.

Toxicity

Essentially nontoxic.

Enemies

Heat, oxygen, freezing temperatures, food-processing, iron, chlorine, mineral oil. [See page 92.]

Personal advice

If you're on a diet high in polyunsaturated oils, you might need additional vitamin E.

Inorganic iron [ferrous sulphate] destroys vitamin E, so the two should not be taken together. If you're using a supplement containing any ferrous sulphate, E should be taken at least eight hours before or after.

Ferrous gluconate, peptonate, citrate, or fumerate [organic iron complexes] do not destroy E.

If you have chlorinated drinking water, you need more vitamin E.

Pregnant or lactating women, as well as those on the pill or taking hormones, need increased vitamin E.

I advise women going through menopause to increase their E intake.

Folic Acid [Folacin]

Facts

Water soluble, another member of the B complex.
Measured in micrograms [mcg.].
Essential to the formation of red blood cells.
Aid in protein metabolism.
The official Recommended Daily Dietary Allowance for adults is 200 mcg.
Important for the production of nucleic acids [RNA and DNA].
Essential for division of body cells.
Needed for utilisation of sugar and amino acids.
Can be destroyed by being stored, unprotected, n temperature for extended time periods.

What it can do for you

Improve lactation.
Protect against intestinal parasites and food poisoning.
Promote healthier-looking skin.
Act as an analgesic for pain.
May delay hair greying when used in conjunction with pantothenic acid and PABA.
Increase appetite, if you are debilitated [run down].
Act as a preventive for canker sores.
Help ward off anaemia.

Deficiency disease

Nutritional macrocytic anaemia.

Best natural sources

Deep-green leafy vegetables, carrots, tortula yeast, liver, egg yolk, melon, apricots, pumpkins, avocados, beans, whole wheat and dark rye flour.

Supplements

Usually supplied in 200-mcg. and 400-mcg. strengths. Strengths of 1 mg. [1,000 mcg.] are available by prescription only.

200 mcg. are sometimes supplied in B-complex formulas, but often only 100 mcg. [Check labels.]

Daily doses most often used are 200 mcg. to 5 mg.

Toxicity

No known toxic effects, though a few people experience allergic skin reactions.

Enemies

Water, sulpha drugs, sunlight, oestrogen, food processing [especially boiling], heat. [See page 92.]

Personal advice

If you are a heavy drinker, it is advisable to increase your folic acid intake.

High vitamin-C intake increases excretion of folic acid, and anyone taking more than 2 g. of C should probably up his folic acid.

If you are on Dilantin or take oestrogens, sulphonamides, phenobarbitone, or aspirin, I suggest increasing folic acid.

I've found that many people taking 1 to 5 mg. daily, for a short period of time, have reversed several types of skin discolouration. If this is a problem to you, it's worth checking out a nutritionally orientated doctor about the possibility.

If you are getting sick, or fighting an illness, make sure your stress supplement has ample folic acid. When folic acid is deficient, so are your antibodies.

Inositol

Facts

Water soluble, another member of the B complex, and a lipotropic.

Measured in milligrams [mg.].

Combines with choline to form lecithin.

Metabolises fats and cholesterol.

Daily dietary allowances have not yet been established, but the average healthy adult gets approximately 1 g. a day.

Like choline, it has been found important in nourishing brain cells.

What it can do for you

Help lower cholesterol levels.

Promote healthy hair — aid in preventing fall-out.

Help in preventing eczema.

Aid in redistribution of body fat.

Deficiency disease

Eczema.

Best natural sources

Liver, brewer's yeast, dried lima beans, beef brains and heart, cantaloupe, grapefruit, raisins, wheat germ, unrefined molasses, peanuts, cabbage.

Supplements

As with choline, six soyabean-based lecithin capsules contain approximately 244 mg. each of inositol and choline.

Available in lecithin powders that mix well with liquids. Most B-complex supplements contain approximately 100 mg. of choline and inositol.

Daily doses most often used are 250 to 500 mg.

Toxicity

No known toxic effects.

Enemies

Water, sulpha drugs, oestrogen, food processing, alcohol, and coffee. [See page 92.]

Personal advice

Take inositol with choline and your other B vitamins.

If you are a heavy coffee drinker, you probably need supplemental inositol.

If you take lecithin, I advise a supplement of chelated calcium to keep your phosphorus and calcium in balance, as both inositol and choline seem to raise phosphorus levels.

A good way to maximise the effectiveness of your vitamin E is to get enough inositol and choline.

Vitamin K [Menadione]

Facts

Not available in the United Kingdom.
Fat soluble.
Usually measured in micrograms [mcg.].
There is a trio of K vitamins, K1 and K2 can be formed by natural bacteria in the intestines. K3 is a synthetic.
No dietary allowance has yet been established.
Essential in the formation of prothrombin, a blood-clotting chemical.

What it can do for you

Help in preventing internal bleeding and haemorrhages.
Aid in reducing excessive menstrual flow.
Promote proper blood clotting.

Deficiency disease

Celiac disease, colitis.

Best natural sources

Yoghurt, alfalfa, egg yolk, safflower oil, soyabean oil, fish liver oils, kelp, leafy green vegetables.

Supplements

The abundance of natural vitamin K generally makes supplementation unnecessary.

It is not included ordinarily in multiple-vitamin capsules.

Toxicity

More than 500 mcg. of synthetic vitamin K is not recommended.

Enemies

X-rays and radiation, frozen foods, aspirin, air pollution, mineral oil. [See page 92.]

Personal advice

Excessive diarrhoea can be a symptom of vitamin-K deficiency, but before self-supplementing, see a doctor.

Yoghurt is your best defence against a vitamin-K deficiency.

If you have nosebleeds often, try increasing your K through natural food sources. Alfalfa tablets might help.

Nicotinamide [Nicotinic Acid, Niacinamide, Niacin]

Facts

Water soluble and a member of the B-complex family, known as B3.

Usually measured in milligrams [mg].

Using the amino acid tryptophan, the body can manufacture its own niacin.

A person whose body is deficient in B1, B2, and B6 will not be able to produce niacin from tryptophan.

Lack of niacin can bring about negative personality changes.

The RDA, according to the National Research Council, is 12 to 18 mg. for adults.

Essential for synthesis of sex hormones [oestrogen, progesterone, testosterone], as well as cortisone, thyroxin, and insulin.

Necessary for healthy nervous system and brain function.

Niacinamide is more generally used since it minimises the flushing and itching of the skin that frequently occurs with the nicotinic acid form of niacin. [The flush, by the way, is not serious and usually disappears in about twenty minutes.]

What it can do for you

Aid in promoting a healthy digestive system, alleviate gastro-intestinal disturbances.

Give you healthier-looking skin.

Help prevent and ease severity of migraine headaches.

Increase circulation and reduce high blood pressure.

Ease some attacks of diarrhoea.

Reduce the unpleasant symptoms of vertigo in Ménière's syndrome.

Increase energy through proper utilisation of food.

Help eliminate canker sores and, often, bad breath.

Reduce cholesterol.

Deficiency disease

Pellagra.

Best natural sources

Liver, lean meat, whole wheat products, brewer's yeast, kidney, wheat germ, fish, eggs, roasted peanuts, the white meat of poultry, avocados, dates, figs, prunes.

Supplements

Available as niacin and niacinamide. [The only difference is that niacin — nicotinic acid — might cause flushing and niacinamide — nicotinamide — will not. If you prefer niacin, you can minimise the flushing by taking your pill on a full stomach or with an equivalent amount of inositol.]

Usually found in 50 to 100-mg. doses in pill and powder form.

50 to 100 mg. are ordinarily included in the better B-complex formulas and multivitamin preparations. [Check labels.]

Toxicity

Essentially nontoxic, except for side effects resulting from doses above 100 mg.

Some sensitive individuals might experience burning or itching skin.

Do not give to animals, especially dogs.

Enemies

Water, sulpha drugs, alcohol, food-processing techniques, sleeping pills, oestrogen. [See page 92.]

Personal advice

If you're taking antibiotics and suddenly find your niacin flushes becoming severe, don't be alarmed.

It's quite common. You'll probably be more comfortable if you switch to niacinamide.

If you have a cholesterol problem, increasing your niacin intake can help.

Skin that is particularly sensitive to sunlight is often an early indicator of niacin deficiency.

Do not give your pets large doses of niacin. It can cause flushing and sweating, greatly distressing the animal and you.

Vitamin P [C Complex, Citrus Bioflavonoids, Rutin, Hesperidin]

Facts

Water soluble and composed of citrin, rutin, and hesperidin, as well as flavones and flavonals.

Usually measured in milligrams [mg.].

Necessary for the proper function and absorption of vitamin C.

Flavonoids are the substances that provide that yellow and orange colour in citrus foods.

Also called the capillary permeability factor. [P stands for permeability.] The prime function of bioflavonoids is to increase capillary strength and regulate absorption.

Aids vitamin C in keeping connective tissues healthy.

No daily allowance has been established, but most nutritionists agree that for every 500 mg. of vitamin C you should have at least 100 mg. of bioflavonoids.

Works synergistically with vitamin C.

What it can do for you

Prevent vitamin C from being destroyed by oxidation.

Strengthen the walls of capillaries, thereby preventing bruising.

Help build resistance to infection.

Aid in preventing and healing bleeding gums.

Increase the effectiveness of vitamin C.
Help in the treatment of oedema and dizziness due to disease of the inner ear.

Deficiency disease

Capillary fragility.

Best natural sources

The white skin and segment part of citrus fruit — lemons, oranges, grapefruit. Also in apricots, buckwheat, blackberries, cherries and rose hips.

Supplements

Available usually in a C complex or by itself. Most often there are 500 mg. of bioflavonoids to 50 mg. of rutin and hesperidin. [If the ratio of rutin and hesperidin is not equal, it should be twice as much rutin.]
All C supplements work better with bioflavonoids.
Most common doses of rutin and hesperidin are 100 mg. three times a day.

Toxicity

No known toxicity.

Enemies

Menopausal women can usually find some effective relief from hot flushes with an increase in bioflavonoids taken in conjunction with vitamin C.

If your gums bleed frequently when you brush your teeth, make sure you're getting enough rutin and hesperidin.

Anyone with a tendency to bruise easily will benefit from a C supplement with bioflavonoids, rutin, and hesperidin.

PABA [Para-aminobenzoic Acid]

Facts

Water soluble, one of the newer members of the B-complex family.

Usually measured in milligrams [mg.].

Can be synthesised in the body.

No RDA has yet been established.

Helps form folic acid and is important in the utilisation of protein.

Has important sun-screening properties.

Helps in the assimilation — and therefore the effectiveness — of pantothenic acid.

In experiments with animals, it has worked with pantothenic acid to restore grey hair to its natural colour.

What it can do for you

Helps to alleviate the pain of rheumatism and arthritis.

Used as an ointment it can protect against sunburn.

Reduce the pain of burns.

Keep skin healthy and smooth.

Help in delaying wrinkles.

Help to restore natural colour to hair.

Deficiency disease

Eczema.

Best natural sources

Liver, brewer's yeast, kidney, whole grains, rice, bran, wheat germ and molasses.

Supplements

30 to 100 mg. are often included in good B-complex capsules as well as high-quality multivitamins.

Available in 30 to 1,000-mg. strengths in regular and time-release form.

Doses most often used are 30 to 100 mg. three times a day.

Toxicity

No known toxic effects, but long-term programmes of high dosages are not recommended.

Symptoms that might indicate an oversupply of PABA are usually nausea and vomiting.

Enemies

Water, sulpha drugs, food-processing techniques
alcohol, oestrogen. [See page 92.]

Personal advice

Some people claim that the combination of folic
acid and PABA has returned their greying hair to
its natural colour. It has worked on animals, so it
is certainly worth a try for anyone looking for an
alternative to hair dye. For this purpose, 1,000
mg. [time release] daily for six days a week is a
viable regimen.

If you tend to burn easily in the sun, use PABA
as a protective ointment.

Many Hollywood celebrities I know use PABA
to prevent wrinkles. It doesn't eliminate them
but it certainly seems to keep them at bay for
some people.

If you are taking penicillin, or any sulpha drug
your PABA intake sould be increased through natu
ral foods or supplements.

Introducing
Minerals

The top six minerals are; calcium, iodine, iron, magnesium, phosphorus, and zinc. Although about eighteen known minerals are required for body maintenance and regulatory functions, Recommended Daily Dietary Allowances (RDA) have only been established for six — calcium, iodine, iron, magnesium, phosphorus, and zinc.

The active minerals in your body are: calcium, chlorine, chromium, cobalt, copper, fluorine, iodine, iron, magnesium, manganese, molybdenum, phosphorus, potassium, selenium, sodium, sulphur, vanadium, and zinc.

Your Body Needs vitamins *and* **minerals**

Vitamins alone are not enough. As important as vitamins are, they can do nothing for you without minerals. I like to call minerals the Cinderellas of the nutrition world, because though very few people are aware of it, vitamins cannot function, cannot be assimilated, without the aids of minerals. And though the body can synthesize some vitamins, it cannot manufacture a *single* mineral.

The ABZ of Minerals

Calcium

Facts

There is more calcium in the body than any other mineral.

Calcium and phosphorus work together for healthy bones and teeth.

Calcium and magnesium work together for cardiovascular health.

Almost all of the body's calcium [two to three pounds] is found in the bones and teeth.

20 percent of an adult's bone calcium is reabsorbed and replaced every year. [New bone cells form as old ones break down.]

Calcium must exist in a two-to-one relationship with phosphorus.

In order for calcium to be absorbed, the body must have sufficient vitamin D.

For adults, 800 to 1,200 mg. is the RDA.

Calcium and iron are the two minerals most deficient in a woman's diet.

What it can do for you

Maintain strong bones and healthy teeth.
Keep your heart beating regularly.
Alleviate insomnia.
Help metabolise your body's iron.
Aid your nervous system, especially in impulse transmission.

Deficiency disease

Rickets, osteomalacia, osteoporosis.

Best natural sources

Milk and milk products, all cheeses, soyabeans, sardines, salmon, peanuts, walnuts, sunflower seeds, dried beans, green vegetables.

Supplements

Most often available on 100- to 500-mg. tablets.

Bonemeal is a fairly common supplement, and a good source of the mineral though some people find calcium gluconate [a vegetarian source] or calcium lactate [a milk sugar derivative] easier to absorb. [Gluconate is more potent than lactate.]

The best form is chelated calcium tablets.

Many good multivitamin and mineral preparations include calcium.

When combined with magnesium, the ratio should be twice as much calcium as magnesium. Dolomite is a natural form of calcium and magnesium, and no vitamin D is needed for assimilation. Five dolomite tablets are equivalent to 750 mg. of calcium.

Doses most often used are 800 to 2,000 mg. per day.

Toxicity

Excessive daily intake of over 2,000 mg. might lead to hypercalcemia.

Enemies

Large quantities of fat, oxalic acid [found in chocolate and rhubarb], and phytic acid [found in grains] are capable of preventing proper calcium absorption.

Personal advice

If you are afflicted with backaches, dolomite, chelated calcium, or bonemeal supplements might help.

Menstrual-cramp sufferers can often find relief by increasing their calcium intake.

Teenagers who suffer from "growing pains" will usually find that they disappear with an increase in calcium consumption.

Hypoglycaemics could use more calcium.

Chlorine

Facts

Regulates the blood's alkaline-acid balance.

Works with sodium and potassium in a compound form.

Aids in the cleaning of body wastes by helping the liver to function.

No dietary allowance has been established, but if your daily salt intake is average, you are getting enough.

What it can do for you

Aid in digestion.
Help keep you limber.

Deficiency disease

Loss of hair and teeth.

Best natural sources

Table salt, kelp, olives

Supplements

Most good multimineral preparations include it.

Toxicity

Over 15g. can cause unpleasant side effects.

Personal advice

If you have chlorine in your drinking water, you aren't getting all the vitamin E you think. [Chlorinated water destroys vitamin E.]

Anyone who drinks chlorinated water would be well advised to eat yoghurt — a good way to replace the intestinal bacteria the chlorine destroys.

Chromium

Facts

Works with insulin in the metabolism of sugar.
Helps bring protein to where it's needed.
No official dietary allowance has been established, but 90 mcg. is an average adult intake.
As you get older, you retain less chromium in your body.

What it can do for you

Aid growth.
Help prevent and lower high blood pressure.

Works as a deterrent for diabetes.

Deficiency disease

A suspected factor in arteriosclerosis and diabetes.

Best natural sources

Meat, shellfish, chicken, corn oil, clams, brewer's yeast.

Supplements

May be found in the better multimineral preparations.

Toxicity

No known toxicity.

Personal advice

If you are low in chromium (a hair analysis would show this) you might try a zinc supplement. For some reason, chelated zinc seems to substitute well for deficient chromium.

Cobalt

Facts

A mineral that is part of vitamin B_{12}.

Usually measured in micrograms [mcg.].
Essential for red blood cells.
Must be obtained from food sources.
No daily allowance has been set for this mineral,
and only very small amounts are necessary in the diet
[usually no more than 8 mcg.].

What it can do for you

Stave off anaemia.

Deficiency disease

Anaemia.

Best natural sources

Meat, kidney, liver, milk, oysters, clams.

Supplements

Rarely found in supplement form.

Toxicity

No known toxicity.

Enemies

Whatever is antagonistic to B_{12}.

Personal advice

If you're a strict vegetarian, you are much more likely to be deficient in this mineral than someone who includes meat and shellfish in his or her diet.

Copper

Facts

Required to convert the body's iron into haemoglobin.

Can reach the bloodstream fifteen minutes after ingestion.

Makes the amino acid tyrosine usable, allowing it to work as the pigmenting factor for hair and skin.

Present in cigarettes, birth-control pills, and automobile pollution.

Essential for the utilisation of vitamin C.

The RDA has not been set by the National Research Council, but 2 mg. for adults is suggested.

What it can do for you

Keep your energy up by aiding in effective iron absorption.

Deficiency disease

Anaemia, edema.

Best natural sources

Dried beans, peas, whole wheat, prunes, calf and beef liver, shrimp, and most seafood.

Supplements

Usually available in multivitamin and mineral supplements in 2-mg. doses.

Toxicity

Rare.

Enemies

Not easily destroyed.

Personal advice

As essential as copper is, I rarely suggest special supplementation. An excess seems to lower zinc level and produce insomnia, hair loss, irregular menses, and depression.

If you eat enough whole-grain products, and fresh green leafy vegetables, as well as liver, you don't have to worry about your copper intake.

Fluorine

Facts

Part of the synthetic compound sodium fluoride [the type added to drinking water] and calcium fluoride [a natural substance].

Decreases chances of dental caries, though too much can discolour teeth.

No RDA has been established, but most people get about 1 mg. daily from fluoridated drinking water.

What it can do for you

Reduce tooth decay.
Strengthen bones.

Deficiency disease

Tooth decay.

Best natural sources

Fluoridated drinking water, seafoods, and gelatin.

Supplements

No ordinarily found in multimineral supplements.

Toxicity

20 to 80 mg. per day.

Enemies

Aluminium salts of fluorine.

Personal advice

Don't take additional fluoride unless it is prescribed by a physician or dentist.

Iodine [Iodide]

Facts

Two-thirds of the body's iodine is in the thyroid
gland.

Since the thyroid gland controls metabolism, and
iodine influences the thyroid, an under-supply of this
mineral can result in slow mental reaction, weight
gain, and lack of energy.

The RDA, as established by the National
Research Council, is 80 to 150 mcg. for adults
[1 mcg. per kilogram of body weight] and 125
to 150 mcg. for pregnant and lactating women
respectively.

What it can do for you

Help you with dieting by burning excess fat.
Promote proper growth.
Give you more energy.
Improve mental alacrity.
Promote healthy hair, nails, skin, and teeth.

Deficiency disease

Goitre, hypothyroidism.

Best natural sources

Kelp, vegetables grown in iodine-rich soil, onions, and all seafood.

Supplements

Available in multimineral and high-potency vitamin supplements in does of 0.15 mg.

Natural kelp is a good source of supplemental iodine.

Toxicity

No known toxicity from natural iodine, though iodine as a drug can be harmful if prescribed incorrectly.

Enemies

Food processing, nutrient-poor soil.

Personal advice

Aside from kelp,and iodine included in multimineral and vitamin preparations, I don't recommend additional supplements unless you're advised by a doctor to take them.

If you use salt and live where iodine-poor soil is common, make sure the salt is iodised.

If you are inclined to eat excessive amounts of raw cabbage, you might *not* be getting the iodine you need, because there are elements in the cabbage that prevent proper utilisation of the iodine. This being the case, you should consider a kelp supplement.

Iron

Facts

Essential and required for life, necessary for the production of haemoglobin [red blood corpuscles], myoglobin [red pigment in muscles], and certain enzymes.

Iron and calcium are the two major dietary deficiencies of women.

Only about 8 percent of your total iron intake is absorbed and actually enters your bloodstream.

An average 150-pound adult has about 4g. of iron in his or her body. Haemoglobin, which accounts for most of the iron, is recycled and reutilised as blood cells are replaced every 120 days. Iron bound to protein [ferritin] is stored in the body, as is tissue iron [present in myoglobin] in very small amounts.

The RDA, according to the National Research Council, is 10 to 18 mg. for adults, and 18 mg. for pregnant and lactating women.

In one month, women lose almost twice as much iron as men.

Copper, cobalt, manganese, and vitamin C are necessary to assimilate iron. Iron is necessary for proper metabolisation of B vitamins.

What it can do for you

Aid growth.
Promote resistance to disease.
Prevent fatigue.
Cure and prevent iron-deficiency anaemia.
Bring back good skin tone.

Deficiency disease

Iron-deficiency anaemia.

Best natural sources

Pork liver, beef kidney, heart and liver, farina, raw
clams, dried peaches, red meat, egg yolks, oysters,
nuts, beans, asparagus, molasses, oatmeal.

Supplements

The most assimilable form of iron is hydrolysed-
protein chelate, which means organic iron that has
been processed for fastest assimilation. This form is
non constipating and easy on sensitive systems.

Ferrous sulphate, inorganic iron, appears in many
vitamin and mineral supplements and can destroy
vitamin E [they should be taken at least eight
hours apart]. Check labels; many formulas contain
ferrous sulphate.

Supplements with organic iron — ferrous gluconate, ferrous fumerate, ferrous citrate, or ferrous peptonate — do not neutralise vitamin E. They are available in a wide variety of does, usually up to 320 mg.

Toxicity

Rare in healthy, normal individuals. Excessive doses, thought, can be a hazard for children.

Enemies

Phosphoproteins in eggs and phytates in unleavened whole wheat reduce iron availability to body.

Personal advice

If you are a woman, I recommend an iron supplement. Check the label on your multivitamin or mineral preparation and see what you are already getting and guide yourself accordingly. [Remember, if the iron in your preparation is ferrous sulphate, you're losing your vitamin E.]

keep your iron supplements out of the reach of children.

Coffee drinkers, as well as tea drinkers, be aware that if you consume large quantities of either beverage you are most likely inhibiting your iron absorption.

Magnesium

Facts

Necessary for calcium and vitamin-C metabolism, as well as that of phosphorus, sodium, and potassium.

Measured in milligrams [mg.]

Essential for effective nerve and muscle functioning.

Important for converting blood sugar into energy.

Known as the antistress mineral.

Alcoholics are usually deficient.

Adults need 300 to 400 mg. daily, slightly more for pregnant and lactating women, according to the US National Research Council.

The human body contains approximately 21g. of magnesium.

What it can do for you

Aid in fighting depression.

Promote a healthier cardiovascular system and help prevent heart attacks.

Keep teeth healthier.

Help prevent calcium deposits, kidney and gallstones.

Bring relief from indigestion.

Deficiency disease

Tremors, nervousness

Best natural sources

Figs, lemons, grapefruit, yellow corn, almonds, nuts, seeds, dark-green vegetables, apples.

Supplements

Dolomite, which has magnesium and calcium in perfect balance [half as much magnesium as calcium], is a fine magnesium supplement.

Available in multivitamin and mineral preparations [best if they are chelated].

Can be purchased as magnesium oxide. 250-mg. strength equals 150 mg. per tablet.

Commonly available in 133.3 -mg. strengths and taken four times a day.

Supplements of magnesium should not be taken after meals, since the mineral does neutralise stomach acidity.

Toxicity

Large amounts, over an extended period of time, can be toxic if your calcium and phosphorous intakes are high

Enemies

Diuretics, alcohol.

Personal advice

If you are a drinker, I suggest you increase your intake of magnesium.

Women who are on the pill or taking oestrogen in any form would be well advised to take larger amounts of magnesium.

If you are a heavy consumer of nuts, seeds, and green vegetables, you probably get ample magnesium — as does anyone who lives in an area with hard water.

Magnesium works best with vitamin A, calcium and phosphorous.

Manganese

Facts

Helps activate enzymes necessary for the body's proper use of biotin, B1, and vitamin C.

Needed for normal bone structure.

Measured in milligrams [mg.].

Important in the formation of thyroxin, the principal hormone of the thyroid gland.

Necessary for the proper digestion and utilisation of food.

No official daily allowance has been set, but 2.5 to 7 mg. is generally accepted to be the average adult requirement.

Important for reproduction and normal central nervous system function.

What it can do for you

Help eliminate fatigue.
Aid in muscle reflexes.
Improve memory.
Reduce nervous irritability.

Deficiency disease

Ataxia.

Best natural sources

Nuts, green leafy vegetables, peas, beets, egg yolks, whole-grain cereals.

Supplements

Most often found in multivitamin and mineral combinations in dosages of 1 to 9 mg.

Toxicity

Rare, except from industrial sources.

Enemies

Large intakes of calcium and phosphorus will inhibit absorption.

Personal advice

If your suffer from recurrent dizziness, you might try adding more manganese to your diet.

I advise absent-minded people, or anyone with memory problems, to make sure they are getting enough of this mineral.

Heavy milk drinkers and meat eaters need increased manganese.

Molybdenum

Facts

Aids in carbohydrate and fat metabolism.

A vital part of the enzyme responsible for iron utilisation.

No dietary allowance has been set, but the estimated daily intake of 45 to 500 mcg. has generally been accepted as the adequate human requirement.

What it can do for you

Help in preventing anaemia.
Promote general well-being.

Deficiency disease

None known.

Best natural sources

Dark-green leafy vegetables, whole grains, legumes.

Supplements

No ordinarily available.

Toxicity

Rare, but 5 to 10 parts per million has been considered toxic.

Personal advice

As important as molybdenum is, there seems no need for supplementation unless all the food you consume comes from nutrient-deficient soil.

Phosphorus

Facts

Present in every cell in the body.

Vitamin D and calcium are essential to proper phosphorus functioning.

Calcium and phosphorus should be balanced two to one to work correctly [twice as much calcium as phosphorus].

Involved in virtually all physiological chemical reactions.

Necessary for normal bone and tooth structure.

Niacin cannot be assimilated without phosphorus.

Important for heart regularity.

Essential for normal kidney functioning.

Needed for the transference of nerve impulses.

The RDA is 800 to 1,200 mg. for adults, the higher levels for pregnant and lactating women.

What it can do for you

Aid in growth and body repair.

Provide energy and vigour by helping in the metabolisation of fats and starches.

Lessen the pain of arthritis.

Promote healthy gums and teeth.

Deficiency disease

Rickets, pyorrhoea.

Best natural sources

Fish, poultry, meat, whole grains, eggs, nuts, seeds.

Supplements

Bonemeal is a fine natural source of phosphorus. [Make sure vitamin D has been added to help assimilation.]

Toxicity

No known toxicity.

Enemies

Too much iron, aluminium, and magnesium can render phosphorus ineffective.

Personal advice

When you get too much phosphorus, you throw off your mineral balance and decrease your calcium. Our diets are usually high in phosphorus — since it does occur in almost every natural food — and therefore calcium deficiencies are frequent. Be aware of this and adjust your diet accordingly.

If you're over forty, you should cut down on your weekly meat consumption and eat more leafy vegetables and drink milk. The reason for this is that after forty our kidneys don't help excrete excess phosphorus, and calcium is again depleted. Be on the lookout for foods preserved with phosphates and consider that as part of your phosphorus intake.

Potassium

Facts

Works with sodium to regulate the body's water balance and normalise heart rhythms. [Potassium works inside the cells, sodium works just outside them.]

Nerve and muscle functions suffer when the sodium-potassium balance is off.

Hypoglycaemia [low blood sugar] causes potassium loss, as does a long fast or severe diarrhoea.

No dietary allowance has been set, but approximately 900 mg. is considered a healthy daily intake.

Both mental and physical stress can lead to a potassium deficiency.

What it can do for you

Aid in clear thinking by sending oxygen to brain.
Help dispose of body wastes.
Assist in reducing blood pressure.
Aid in allergy treatment.

Deficiency disease

Edema, hypoglycaemia.

Best natural sources

Citrus fruits, watercress, all green leafy vegetables, mint leaves, sunflower seeds, bananas, potatoes.

Supplements

In most high-potency multivitamin and multimineral preparations.

Inorganic potassium "salts" are the sulphate [alum], the chloride, the oxide and carbonate. Organic potassium refers to the gluconate, the citrate, the fumerate.

Can be bought separately as potassium gluconate in dosages up to nearly 600 mg.

Toxicity

25 g. of potassium chloride can cause toxicity.

Enemies

Alcohol, coffee, sugar, diuretics.

Personal advice

If you drink large amounts of coffee, you might find that the fatigue you're fighting is due to the potassium loss you're suffering from.

Heavy drinkers and anyone with a hungry sweet tooth should be aware that their potassium levels are probably low.

If you have low blood sugar, you are likely to be losing potassium while retaining water. And if you take a diuretic, you'll lose even more potassium. Watch your diet, increase your green vegetables, and take enough magnesium to regain your mineral balance.

Losing weight on a low-carbohydrate diet might not be the only thing you're losing. Chances are your potassium level is down. Watch out for weakness and poor reflexes.

Selenium

Facts

Vitamin E and selenium are synergistic. This means that the two together are stronger than the sum of the equal parts.

Both vitamin E and selenium are antioxidants, preventing or at least slowing down aging and hardening of tissues through oxidation.

Males appear to have a greater need for selenium. Almost half their body's supply concentrates in the testicles and portions of the seminal ducts adjacent to the prostate gland. Also, selenium is lost in the semen.

No official dietary allowance has been set for this mineral, but the general dosage is between 50 and 100 mcg. It is not advisable to exceed 200 mcg. daily.

What it can do for you

Aid in keeping youthful elasticity in tissues.
Alleviate hot flushes and menopausal distress.
Help in treatment and prevention of dandruff.
Possibly neutralise certain carcinogens and provide protection from some cancers.

Deficiency disease

Premature stamina loss.

Best natural sources

Wheat germ, bran, tuna fish, onions, tomatoes, broccoli.

Supplements

Available in small microgram doses. 25 to 50 mcg. is most often used.

Also available combined with vitamin E and other antioxidants.

Natural foods supply sufficient amounts when eaten regularly.

Toxicity

Doses above 5 parts per million can be toxic.

Enemies

Food-processing techniques.

Personal advice

Selenium was discovered only a little more than twenty years ago. We've just begun to recognise its importance in human nutrition. Until more is known,

I advise taking only moderate supplements.

Sodium

Facts

Sodium and potassium were discovered together and both found to be essential for normal growth.

High intakes of sodium [salt] will result in a depletion of potassium.

Diets high in sodium usually account for many instances of high blood pressure.

There is no official allowance, but a daily single gram of sodium chloride has been suggested for each kilogram of water drunk. Sodium aids in keeping calcium and other minerals in the blood soluble.

What it can do for you

Aid in preventing heat prostration or sunstroke
Help your nerves and muscles function
properly.

Deficiency disease

Impaired carbohydrates digestion, possibly neuralgia.

Best natural sources

Salt, shellfish, carrots, beets, artichokes, dried beef, brains, kidney, bacon.

Supplements

Rarely needed, but if so, kelp is a safe and nutritive supplement.

Toxicity

Over 14 g. of sodium chloride daily can produce toxic effects.

Personal advice

If you think you don't eat much salt, you are probably mistaken.

If you have high blood pressure, cut down on your sodium intake by reading the labels on the foods you buy. Look for *salt*, *sodium*, or the chemical symbol *Na*.

Adding sodium to your diet is as easy as a shake of salt, but subtracting it can be difficult. Avoid luncheon meats, frankfurters, salted cured meats such as ham, bacon, corned beef, as well as condiments — ketchup, chilli sauce, soya sauce, mustard. Don't use baking powder or baking soda in cooking.

Sulphur

Facts

Essential for healthy hair, skin and nails.

Helps maintain oxygen balance necessary for proper brain function.

Works with B-complex vitamins for basic body metabolism, and is part of tissue-building amino acids.

Aids the liver in bile secretion.

No RDA has been set, but a diet sufficient in protein will generally be sufficient in sulphur.

What it can do for you

Tone up skin and make hair more lustrous.
Help fight bacterial infections.

Deficiency disease

None known.

Best natural sources

Lean beef, dried beans, fish, eggs, cabbage.

Supplements

Not readily available as a food supplement.
Can be found in topical ointments and creams for skin problems.

Toxicity

No known toxicity from organic sulphur, but ill effects may occur from large amounts of inorganic sulphur.

Personal advice

If you're getting enough protein in your daily meals,you are, most likely,getting enough sulphur.

Sulphur creams and ointments have been remarkably successful in treating a variety of skin problems. Check the ingredients in the preparation you are now using. There are many fine natural preparations available at healthfood centres.

Vanadium

Facts

Inhibits the formation of cholesterol in blood vessels.

No dietary allowance set.

What it can do for you

Aid in preventing heart attacks.

Deficiency disease

None known.

Best natural sources

Fish.

Supplements

Not available.

Toxicity

Can easily be toxic if taken in synthetic form.

Personal advice

This is not one of the minerals that needs to be supplemented. A good fish dinner will supply you with the vanadium you need.

Zinc

Facts

Zinc acts as a traffic policeman, directing and overseeing the efficient flow of body processes, the maintenance of enzyme system and cells.

Essential for protein synthesis.

Governs the contractibility of muscles.

Helps in the formation of insulin.

Important for blood stability and in maintaining the body's acid-alkaline balance.

Exerts a normalising effect on the prostate and is important in the development of all reproductive organs.

New studies indicate its importance in brain function and the treatment of schizophrenia.

Strong evidence of its requirement for the synthesis of DNA.

The RDA, as set by the U.S. National Research Council, is 15 mg. for adults [slightly higher allowances for pregnant and lactating women].

Excessive sweating can cause a loss of as much as 3 mg. of zinc per day.

Most zinc in foods is lost in processing, or never exists in substantial amount due to nutrient-poor soil.

What it can do for you

Accelerate healing time for internal and external wounds.

Get rid of white spots on the fingernails.

Help eliminate loss of taste.

Aid in the treatment of infertility.

Help avoid prostate problems.

Promote growth and mental alertness.

Help decrease cholesterol deposits.

Deficiency disease

Possibly prostatic hypertrophy [non-cancerous enlargement of the prostate gland], arteriosclerosis.

Best natural sources

Round steak, lamb chops, pork loin, wheat germ, brewer's yeast, pumpkin seeds, eggs, nonfat dry milk, ground mustard.

Supplements

Available in all good multivitamin and multi-mineral preparations.

Can be bought as zinc-sulphate or zinc-gluconate tablets in doses ranging from 15 to over 300 mg. Both zinc sulphate and zinc gluconate seem to be equally effective, but zinc gluconate appears to be more easily tolerated.

Chelated zinc is the best way to take zinc.

Zinc is also available in combination with vitamin C, magnesium, and the B-complex vitamins.

Toxicity

Virtually nontoxic, except when there is an excessive intake and the food ingested has been stored in galvanised containers. Doses over 150 mg. are not recommended.

Personal advice

You need higher intakes of zinc if you are taking large amounts of vitamin B6. This is also true if you are an alcoholic or a diabetic.

Men with prostate problems — and without them — would be well advised to keep their zinc levels up.

I have seen success in cases of impotence with a supplement programme of B6 and zinc.

Elderly people, concerned about senility, might find a zinc and manganese supplement beneficial.

If you are bothered by irregular menses, you might try a zinc supplement before resorting to hormone treatment to establish regularity.

Remember, if you are adding zinc to your diet, you will increase the need for vitamin A. Zinc works best with vitamin A, calcium and phosphorus.

Water

Facts

The simple truth is that this is our most important nutrient. One-half to three-quarters of the body's weight is water.

A human being can live for weeks without food, but only a few days without water.

Water is the basic solvent for all the products of digestion.

Essential for removing wastes.

There is no specific dietary allowance since water loss varies with climate, situations, and individuals, but under ordinary circumstances six glasses daily is considered healthy.

Regulates body temperature.

What it can do for you

Keep all your bodily functions functioning.
Aid in dieting by depressing appetite before meals.
Help prevent constipation.

Deficiency disease

Dehydration.

Best natural sources

Drinking water, juices, fruits, and vegetables.

Supplements

All drinkable liquids can substitute for only daily water requirements.

Toxicity

No known toxicity, but an intake of one and a half gallons [that's sixteen to twenty-four glasses] in about an hour could be dangerous for an adult. It could kill an infant.

Personal advice

I advise six to eight glasses of water daily, to be drunk a half hour before meals, for anyone who's dieting.

If you're running a fever, be sure to drink lots of water to prevent dehydration and to flush system wastes.

If you live in an area where there is hard water, you're probably getting more calcium and magnesium than you think.

DRUGS THAT INDUCE VITAMIN DEFICIENCIES

Three basic mechanisms exist by which drugs induce vitamin deficiencies

A. Impaired vitamin absorption
B. Impaired vitamin utilisation
C. Enhanced vitamin elimination

A. Impairment of vitamin absorption

Drug	Vitamins depleted
Glutethimide	Folic acid
Cholestyramine	A, D, E, K, and B12
Os-Cal-Mone	B6
Mineral Oil	A, D, E, and K
Polysporin, Neo-Sporin, Neo-mycin Mycolog, Neo-Cortef, Cortisporin, Lidosporin, Mycifradin	K, B12, and folic acid
Kanamycin	K and B12
Tetracycline	K, calcium, magnesium, and iron
Chloramphenical	K
Polymyxin	K
Sulphonamides	K
Phazyme	K
Sulphasalazine, Aso-Gantanol	Folic Acid
Colchicine, Colbenemid	B12, A, and potassium
Trifluoperazine	B12
Cortisone	B6, D, C, zinc, and potassium
Cathartic agents	B2, K
Antacids	A and B

B. Impairment of vitamin utilisation

Drug	Vitamins depleted
Coumarins	K
Pro-Banthine, Probital	K
Methotrexate	Folic acid
Triamterene	Folic acid
Pyrimethamine	Folic acid
Trimethoprim	Folic acid
Nitrofurantoin	Folic acid
Phenylbutazone	Folic acid
Aspirin	Folic acid, C, and B1
Indomethacin	B1 and C
Bentyl with Phenobarb, Cantil with Phenobarb, Isordil with phenobarb	K

C. Enhanced vitamin excretion

Drug	Vitamins depleted
Aldactazide, Altactone	Potassium
Isoniazid	B6
Hydralazine	B6
Ser-Ap-Es	B6
Penicillamine	B6
Clorothiazide	Magnesium and potassium
Boric Acid	B2
Bronkotabs, Bronkolixer	K
Chardonna	K

Drugs with Multiple Mechanisms

Drug	Vitamins depleted
Diethylstilbestrol	B6
Anticonvulsants	Folic acid and D
Phenytoin	Folic acid and D
Barbiturates	Folic acid and D
Oral contraceptive steroids	Folic acid, C, and B6
Alcohol	B1, folic acid, and K
Betapar	B6, C, zinc, and potassium

GLOSSARY

absorption: the process by which nutrients are passed into the bloodstream

acetate: a derivative of acetic acid

acid: a water-soluble substance with sour taste

alkali: An acid-neutralising substance (sodium bicarbonate is an alkali used for excess acidity in foods)

Alzheimer's disease: a progressively degenerative disease involved with loss of memory, that new research indicates might be helped with extra choline

amino acids: the organic compounds from which proteins are constructed; there are twenty-two known amino acids, but only nine are indispensable nutrients for man — histidine, isoleucine, leucine, lysine, total S-containing amino acids, total aromatic amino acids, threonine, tryptophan, and valine

antioxidant: a substance that can protect another substance from oxidation; added to food to keep oxygen from changing the food's colour

assimilation: the process whereby nutrients are used by the body and changed into living tissue

bioflavonoids: usually from orange and lemon rinds, these citrus-flavoured compounds needed to maintain healthy blood-vessel walls are widely available in plants, citrus fruits and rose hips; known as vitamin P complex

calciferol: a colourless, odourless crystalline material, insoluble in water; soluble in fats; a synthetic form of vitamin D made by irradiating ergosterol with ultraviolet light

capillary: a minute blood vessel, one of many that connect the arteries and veins

carotene: an orange-yellow pigment occurring in many plants, and capable of being converted into vitamin A in the body

chelation: a process by which mineral substances are bound into organic protein to improve assimilation

collagen: the primary organic constituent of bone cartilage and connective tissue (becomes gelatin through boiling)

diuretic: tending to increase the flow of urine from the body

DNA: deoxyribonucleic acid; the nucleic acid in chromosomes that is part of the chemical basis for hereditary characteristics

enzyme: a protein substance found in living cells that brings about chemical changes; necessary for digestion of food

FDA: Food and Drugs Administration (USA)

hesperidin: part of the C complex

hormone: a substance formed in endocrine organs and transported by body fluids to activate other specially receptive organs

hypolycaemia: a condition caused by abnormally low blood sugar

IU: International Units

lactating: producing milk

laxative: A substance that stimulates evacuation of the bowels

linoleic acid: one of the polyunsaturated fats, a constituent of lecithin; known as vitamin F; indispensable for life, and must be obtained from foods

lipotropic: preventing abnormal or excessive accumulation of fat in the liver

metabolise: to undergo change by physical and chemical changes

toxicity: the quality or condition of being poisonous, harmful or destructive

toxin: an organic poison produced in living or dead organisms

unsaturated fatty acids: most often liquid at room temperature, primarily found in vegetable fats

U.S. RDA: United States Recommended Daily Allowances